Table of Contents

Asthma Testing for Diagnosis and Treatment

1. Introduction to Asthma

1.1. Definition and Epidemiology

1.2. Pathophysiology

2. Clinical Presentation of Asthma

2.1. Symptoms and Signs

2.2. Severity Classification

3. Diagnostic Tests for Asthma

3.1. Spirometry

3.2. Peak Expiratory Flow (PEF)

4. Additional Diagnostic Tools

4.1. Bronchial Provocation Testing

4.2. Allergy Testing

5. Differential Diagnosis of Asthma

5.1. Chronic Obstructive Pulmonary Disease (COPD)

5.2. Heart Failure

6. Treatment Guidelines for Asthma

6.1. Pharmacological Management

6.2. Non-Pharmacological Interventions

7. Asthma Action Plans

8. Monitoring Asthma Control

9. Emerging Technologies in Asthma Diagnosis and Treatment

Diagnostic Tests for Asthma-Like Symptoms

1. Introduction to Asthma-Like Symptoms

2. Importance of Diagnostic Tests

3. Medical History and Physical Examination

4. Pulmonary Function Tests

4.1. Spirometry

4.2. Peak Flow Test

5. Imaging Tests

5.1. Chest X-ray

5.2. CT Scan

6. Allergy Testing

7. Blood Tests

8. Sputum Eosinophil Count

9. Bronchoprovocation Testing

10. Exhaled Nitric Oxide Test

11. Bronchoscopy

12. Other Potential Tests

13. Preparing for Diagnostic Tests

14. Understanding Test Results

15. Common Misconceptions and FAQs

Asthma Testing for Diagnosis and Treatment

1. Introduction to Asthma

Tests for asthma are not only designed to help medical professionals diagnose the disease in individuals but are also crucial to assess how well those who are diagnosed with asthma are improving and how best to manage the disease to prevent exacerbation while maintaining good lung function. Testing for asthma is particularly important in ensuring that children with the disease can still lead normal and active lives. One of the multiple asthma testing techniques, spirometry, assesses how much, how fast, and how forcefully air can be exhaled from the lungs. This test can help determine if the individual has asthma, how well the person takes medications for asthma, and help determine occupational asthma. Impulse oscillometry helps assess the severity of asthma through measuring how large airways are. Other techniques include the FeNO test, methacholine challenge, asthma skin prick test, and sputum, blood, or urine cell test.

Among chronic diseases, asthma is widely prevalent, affecting about 334 million people as of 2010. Asthma was responsible for 250,000 deaths in 2009, which led to costs of about an average of $3000. While asthma is more frequently diagnosed during childhood, all individuals are susceptible to being diagnosed at any age of their life. Public health is heavily impacted by asthma, as individuals are inhibited from participating in physical activity, attending school, and attending work. Symptoms of asthma include a tight feeling in the chest and shortness of breath.

Attacks of asthma have several triggers, including but not limited to smoke, allergens, and low air temperatures. The disease is diagnosed via a person's medical history and does not have a cure. The management of asthma includes environmental modifications, using medications such as chest inhalers, and preventing exacerbation of the disease and improving lung function via a plethora of tests and techniques.

1.1. Definition and Epidemiology

When patients with chronic cough and asthma are evaluated for chronic cough or persistent wheezing and persistent dry cough over many weeks, who have cough exacerbated on exposure to irritants such as perfume or cologne, or who have long, episodic coughing fits that are at their most severe in cold dry weather, then it is important to measure the histograms for testing at baseline, if possible, and compare them with those obtained following selective bronchodilator use. Statistical comparisons may allow a distinction to be made between reversible and fixed airway obstruction in adults. Active acute respiratory symptoms present during testing will usually cause airway hyperresponsiveness immediately postexercise in children and flare within 24 to 48 hours when tested by methacholine, histamine, exercise, or other forms of indirect airways challenge testing.

Asthma is a complex but very common disease affecting all ages and is defined by three primary characteristics: airway inflammation, airway hyperresponsiveness, and reversible airflow obstruction. It is more prevalent in children than in adults, more common in women than in men, and has significant variability in frequency, severity, and distribution within and between developed and developing countries. The World Health Organization has defined asthma as "a serious complex, chronic disease of the airways that is characterized by variable and recurring symptoms, airflow obstruction, bronchospasm, dyspnea, and variable extrapulmonary features of airway hyperresponsiveness syndrome." Extrapolation from studies conducted in Europe, Canada, and the United States suggests that current patterns of morbidity and asthma-related mortality will worsen. Experts estimate that asthma currently affects over 334 million people worldwide and that as much as 12.7% of the global burden of the disease can be attributed to asthma. Rates of asthma-related emergency room visits and hospitalization are disproportionately higher in women and are most common in children and older adults. The typical treatment under these circumstances is with corticosteroids, but there is no specific diagnosis that can accurately identify and assess cases of adult asthma.

1.2. Pathophysiology

Outcome measurement in asthma can be performed using measurements of airflow such as spirometry and airway hyperresponsiveness, symptoms of airflow limitation, and quality of life assessments of patients. Spirometry assesses airflow limitation, however, is known to be insensitive in detecting mild asthma, in detecting airway changes, and the current level of inflammation. Airway hyperresponsiveness is uneven in its expression and varies in between- and within-patient measurements. Consequently, it may not be enough to identify asthma, especially the milder forms, or to monitor changes in asthma control longitudinally. Furthermore, there is currently no available gold standard for the diagnosis, assessment, and management of asthma. Chronic oral or inhaled steroid treatment can decrease and mask the severity of the airway inflammation and consequently arterial oxygen saturation. Similarly, an inhaled long-acting $\beta2$-agonist bronchodilator may open the airways, thus decreasing any airway narrowing, and consequently flow limitation. In contrast, the use of preventive asthma therapy, such as inhaled corticosteroids, or reliever medication may decrease a patient's symptoms and bronchoconstriction and in the absence of diagnostic testing, does not allow for a definitive diagnosis or evaluation of their asthma. A diagnostic testing profile is presented in Figure 1. Asthma is a syndrome classically defined by symptoms and supported by physiologic measurements of variable expiratory airflow limitation from a relative site of obstruction in the trachea, bronchi, and bronchioles and with increased thoracic gas volume due to air trapping.

Asthma is a complex heterogeneous syndrome characterized by variable respiratory symptoms such as wheeze, shortness of breath, chest tightness, and cough, airflow limitation, and airway hyperresponsiveness. The underlying pathophysiology includes various processes such as inflammation, airway wall remodeling, and airway hyperactivity. Inflammation, involving mainly eosinophils and T-helper cells, increases the vascular permeability which causes edema, mucus production, and exacerbates bronchoconstriction, contributing to airway limitation in asthma. Some individuals, especially those with severe asthma, have airway remodeling with thickening of the airway basement membrane, hypertrophy, and hyperplasia of the airway smooth muscle layer, which can limit airflow in these patients. Airway hyperresponsiveness causes the airways to constrict more vigorously to a variety of external and endogenous agents compared to non-asthmatics. Furthermore, airway inflammation, remodeling, and hyperactivity are also thought to contribute to chronic airway limitation and to the association of asthma with fixed airway limitation or chronic obstructive pulmonary disease.

2. Clinical Presentation of Asthma

The four most common symptoms that patients with asthma tend to have in the general practice setups, which based on the data from The International Study of Asthma and Allergies in Childhood (ISAAC) study are: breathlessness, wheezing, chest tightness, and cough. These symptoms might, however, reduce the quality of life of an individual. The signs and symptoms of asthma can be classified into major and minor signs and symptoms, these are presented in Table 1. Several factors expose an individual to have increased chances of having asthma, for example, chronic exposure to dust or allergic reaction, occupational exposure in the work environment, smoking, use of bronchodilators for more than three days, presence of rhinitis, eczema, and atopy. Blood eosinophils count of less than 600 indicates fewer chances of having a diagnosis of asthma. Some clinical presentations of asthma are shown in Table 1 below and should caution the health provider to consider the management of the condition.

In general, the clinical manifestations of asthma vary from patient to patient, but most patients present the following signs and symptoms. Typically, the presence of one or more of these predictive factors often leads to the diagnosis of asthma initiation of diagnostic procedure, though the sensitivity and specificity of the tests are relatively low. This section presents the major clinical presentation of asthma that triggers the need for asthma diagnostic tests and initiation of treatment.

6.2. Non-Pharmacological Interventions

A two-pronged approach can assist in asthma management, pharmacological interventions and non-pharmacological interventions. The non-pharmacological interventions are lifestyle interventions and control of environmental factors from the outset. Lifestyle modifications encompass a set of physical activities recommended for healthy living, that includes an exercise schedule, food habits, and smoking cessation methods. The patient is also educated to control stress and anxiety by adopting yoga, deep breathing exercises, musical therapy, and accepting parental support. Identifying the patient as allergic 117 Environmental control measures are identifying probable allergens with the intention of reducing the likelihood to come in contact with these allergens. This helps to decrease the frequency of the asthma triggers and subsequently the number of episodes can be reduced.

The non-pharmacological interventions for asthma include lifestyle modifications and environmental control measures. Effective diagnosis can guide the clinicians to plan the treatment as per the need of the patient. Thorough control of these aspects helps in reducing the respiratory symptoms during this season. The emergency hospital visits can also be decreased significantly by reducing the contact with a specific allergen or the occupational exposure which can result in asthma worsening. The identification of the allergen/trigger possibly responsible for the asthma symptoms becomes indispensable for its

2.1. Symptoms and Signs

Several symptoms and signs suggest a diagnosis of asthma: symptoms occur or worsen in response to triggers such as exercise, allergens, airborne irritants, medicines, smoke (including primarily passive smoke); symptoms are chronic or recur at least intermittently; positive family history; coexisting conditions associated with an increased risk of developing asthma (see chapter 6.2). In patients consulting a physician, key symptoms include prolonged cough, ongoing symptoms or recurrent wheeze (especially nocturnal), dyspnoea or chest tightness during exercise, and respiratory symptoms that interfere with normal daily activities. However, such symptoms might also indicate other conditions including infection, COPD, and cystic fibrosis. Given the above, more objective tests (see chapter 6 of the strategy) are almost always needed to diagnose asthma. If left untreated, new onset asthma is frequently progressive. Prompt and sustained treatment can halt the course to chronic asthma in some, but not all, children. Early recognition and intervention might be particularly important in these patients. Whether new onset asthma can be cured by treatment is less certain.

Asthma symptoms can be intermittent and are often experienced in response to various triggers (e.g., allergens, irritants). Respiratory symptoms of asthma are: cough (with/without sputum), wheeze, shortness of breath, and chest tightness. In many cases, periodic wheezing or chronic cough are the only symptoms. Disturbed sleep is common, and many people experience relief from symptoms during the day. Wheezing or cough triggered by the coexistence of rhinitis could suggest asthma if there is no strong evidence for another diagnosis, the wheezes occur in the chest, asthma symptoms have anteceded the onset of rhinitis, and there is concomitant bronchoscopic evidence of asthma.

2.2. Severity Classification

The classification of asthma severity will be based on the presence and frequency of day symptoms, the frequency of nighttime and early morning symptoms, the need for rescue treatment with short-acting b2 agonists (SABA), limitation in daily physical activity, lung function, eNO, and the future risk of adverse events. The approach to asthma patients will also depend on the classification of the severity of the disease, starting from a detailed phenotyping to achieve a personalized approach. In the management step, asthma severity has been divided into four different levels. Briefly, intermittent asthma is classified as level 1, mild asthma as level 2, moderate asthma as level 3, and finally, severe asthma as level 4.

Patients with suspected asthma should be thoroughly evaluated and classified after the formulaic approach, based on specific history and a complete diagnostic workup which will allow the exclusion of any asthma mimickers. The evaluation of the disease may help in defining the range of the different objective tests to be performed, with lung function, i.e., including both spirometry and bronchial reversibility, being the cornerstone diagnostic evaluation. Atopic and non-atopic conditions will need to be differentiated as well, in order to choose the optimal therapeutic pathway.

3. Diagnostic Tests for Asthma

Measure the variability of peak expiratory flow and graph it for display over time, days or weeks, to see the pattern of different responses in asthma. History taking usually tells the physician when to consider this form of testing, either to confirm if a diagnosis of asthma reflects the disease, or to evaluate ongoing treated or untreated asthma. It is easily performed and can be useful but, when done in a non-structured way, does not usually show the characteristic of a true pattern of asthma. Most types of unusual variability can occur in several diseases with the ultimate result being asthma, as shown by a good response to anti-inflammatory or bronchodilating medications.

Assess the degree of cough and symptoms of asthma, the degree of airflow obstruction, and response to medication. Spirometry measures breathing volumes and airflow rates at the mouth. There are some parameters that can be worked out from a normal spirogram that are useful for evaluating the response to treatment and the person's fitness for surgery. Airway resistance can be measured in special laboratories. Reflex bronchospasm can be initiated by exercise or by ingestion of some nicotinic agents. Anxiety and bronchospasm do not always relieve themselves merely because the offending stimulus is being removed. The limitations include both harm and not being diagnostic of asthma. They do not establish reversible airway obstruction. They cannot be used in people unable to perform full function tests. They are often normal in people with chronic asthma, and may become positive in people without asthma. When interpreting these tests, the athlete must not be taking medication.

Various instruments and devices are used in confirming or evaluating the diagnosis of asthma. A number of different tests may be appropriate for different circumstances. However, it is important to understand the purpose and value of the tests. Some confirm the diagnosis and give an assessment of severity, others are useful for measuring treatment of asthma. Testing may show that asthma is not present, appear normal or indicate evidence of asthma, reversible airway obstruction, bronchial hyper-responsiveness, bronchodilator response.

3.1. Spirometry

The procedure to perform the test is explained in a dedicated section in the chapter on diagnostic tests. This manuscript will primarily deal with the interpretation of spirometric data for a correct asthma diagnosis and periodic assessment of lung function's improvement or deterioration in response to treatments. Diagnosis and monitoring of occupational or work-related asthma also include serial measurements of lung function. It is essential to integrate the clinical and functional picture with the clinical history and physical examination. In this context, a special role can be played by FeNO and bronchial challenge tests. A normal spirometric function does not rule out a diagnosis of asthma if a significant clinical history is present, and measures of FEV1 variability may help clarify the diagnosis.

Spirometry is strongly recommended as the best test to diagnose asthma when the diagnosis is not clear from the symptoms and medical history. Spirometry is also used to assess how well treatment is working, check whether asthma symptoms are related to exercise, and diagnose other conditions that could be causing asthma-like symptoms. A flow-volume loop is a graphical representation of airflow plotted as a function of lung volume. An upper airway obstruction typically presents as a concave scorpion tail configuration on a flow-volume loop, which allows accurate discrimination between extrathoracic and intrathoracic airway pathology. Spirometry provides measures of dynamic lung volumes and capacities useful to distinguish asthma from COPD and between other obstructive lung diseases. These measurements are: forced vital capacity (FVC), forced expiratory volume in 1 second (FEV1), forced expiratory flow between 25% and 75% of FVC (FEF25-75% or Mid-FEF), and FEV1/FVC, and may also provide additional relevant information such as bronchodilator response and bronchial hyperresponsiveness.

3.2. Peak Expiratory Flow (PEF)

Potential contributing factors to variability in PEF measurements result from the instruments themselves, variables used in the population studies, time of measurement, and result interpretation. The high variations of the PEF occur amongst individuals and in the same person. Several factors directly included in this variation are related to the individual's characteristics, such as age, sex, weight, and height. The variables related to the instrument variation, however, include the intensity of the blow, the calibration of the equipment, and the motivation of the patient. Factors like height, sex, and age directly influence PEF measurements while others indirectly do so. It is important to normalize PEF for age, sex, and height. Appropriate measurement technique is essential.

Peak Expiratory Flow (PEF) testing. PEF is the maximum flow rate obtained during expiration and is assessed during a person's maximum forced expiration after a full inspiration. The best flow rate is obtained from a single forced expiration and then repeated three times to obtain the best effort. During acute exacerbation, the forced maneuver might increase symptoms, and a lower value is sometimes obtained due to fatigue. The flow is influenced by the patient's effort; if the patient does not perform it correctly, the value is low. However, if the patient practices, repeat sessions can be influenced by learning and improvement in results, leading to higher values. PEF measurements assess airway obstruction and can detect changes, as well as assess airway hyperresponsiveness. This test is important in asthmatic patients since they recognize and characterize the disease. As a monitoring test, it is utilized to assist in making decisions to adjust treatment.

4. Additional Diagnostic Tools

The assessment of airway inflammation should be considered in the diagnostic assessment of asthma. This would normally be assessed by obtaining a blood eosinophil count, FENO or sputum eosinophil count. All of these are surrogates for an induced sputum count - in which patients are required to provide expectorated sputum for quantification of eosinophils. Elevated levels in the absence of significant symptoms would fit the asthma picture much more than ACE and an elevated AEC resulting in eosinophil mediated tissue damage. Allergy testing, including skin prick testing and allergen-specific IgE measurement, is a useful component of asthma diagnosis. Awareness of the various tests is essential for any clinician involved in the evaluation and diagnosis of suspected asthma.

Several additional diagnostic tools can be useful in augmenting the comprehensive diagnostic evaluation of asthma. The exercise challenge test demonstrates levels of exercise that do not trigger symptoms. This is a particularly useful test, as active asthma (albeit controlled) is likely to have some level of underlying airway hypersensitivity. The methacholine, mannitol or histamine provocation test produces the concentration of the drug required to provoke a 20% fall in airway calibre (the PD20 – provocative dose falling within the last 20% of the dose-response curve). An individual with underlying bronchial hyperresponsiveness (common in asthma), will reach this level at a significantly lower concentration of the drug than an age matched control (Table 2). Provocation testing to mannitol has been recommended as it is quicker, better tolerated, and safer than the indirect challenges based on cholinergic agonists. The test can be ordered through either children's or adult's hospitals; the test procedure is available from National Asthma Council of Australia.

Asthma is a highly prevalent disease with an extensive variability in presentation and severity. The pathophysiologic hallmark of asthma is AHR, which has been known since the 17th century. The body of evidence from experts in the field indicates that AHR is present in a significant majority of asthmatics and that the degree of AHR is correlated with the severity of this condition. However, AHR may also be present in other types of lung diseases, such as chronic obstructive pulmonary disease (COPD), allergic bronchopulmonary aspergillosis, and even in non-respiratory conditions, including systemic sclerosis and bronchiectasis. Therefore, the present definition of asthma states that this condition is characterized by AHR and inflammation, which is generally present in most individuals. It is possible that asthmatics could have isolated inflammation (in the absence of AHR) or AHR without airway inflammation, but those are rare findings. The aim of bronchial provocation testing is to induce bronchoconstriction, which is usually characterized by a fall in forced expiratory volume in one second (FEV1) from baseline of 20% or higher.

One of the current trends in the phenotyping of asthma is to identify treatable traits. Treatable traits include airway hyperresponsiveness (AHR), airway inflammation, and airway obstruction in a wide variability of phenotypes and genotypes. The use of bronchial provocation testing has been suggested for both the diagnosis and treatment of asthma, despite the usefulness of this provocative agent, which can distinguish between poorly controlled asthmatics and other types of respiratory disorders. The use of proper bronchial provocation could result in a new way of phenotyping asthma.

4.2. Allergy Testing

Skin testing should be used as a complementary method to blood testing if the blood test is negative but the clinical history strongly suggests allergic asthma. If there is strong evidence of allergic asthma at the beginning (e.g. only complaints during certain seasons, a clear relationship between smoldering or atopy in childhood and the onset of asthma), skin testing may be sufficient. Testing for sensitization without a clear need fails to add value to the diagnostic process of asthma. A proven allergy is required to initiate targeted treatment to reduce and ideally eliminate exposure to allergens. For example, for elderly women with asthma, in general, it is doubtful whether an allergy test is carried out. Symptomatic therapy with substances that block or attempt to inhibit inflammatory pathways initiates anti-inflammatory therapy.

The immune system is responsible for the body's defense against harmful substances. If your immune system reacts disproportionately to harmless proteins, an allergy can develop. The allergic reactions of the immune system can trigger typical symptoms such as hay fever, skin redness or itching, asthma, and vomiting and diarrhea. If the asthma was caused by an allergy, this should be detected in test methods in the blood and in the skin (allergy test). Allergy testing is used to identify the allergen to which the allergic person has unnecessarily developed specific IgE antibodies. The detection of these antibodies in the blood (specific IgE) is currently preferred. This avoids unnecessary direct contact with the allergen in the skin and subjective misinterpretation.

5. Differential Diagnosis of Asthma

Patients with symptoms of cough, wheeze, chest tightness or shortness of breath will be asked if they experience symptoms daily, almost daily or with decreasing frequency, as well as if they are associated with specific allergens. Recent guidance suggests that if symptoms are present on a daily basis, asthma is likely present, and testing should focus on confirming the diagnosis. Smoking for a long period without excess phlegm production is six times more likely to be from pulmonary parenchymal damage instead of airflow obstruction, suggesting COPD versus earlier-onset asthma. Physical examination to evaluate for other airway diseases, such as chronic obstructive pulmonary disease (COPD), vocal cord dysfunction or chronic systolic heart failure (e.g., accessory muscle use, tripodding, speaking in short sentences, tachypnea, diaphoresis, delayed capillary refill, edema), may help exclude other chronic lung diseases.

The differential diagnosis of asthma involves excluding other conditions that can present in similar manners, such as an upper airway obstruction like subglottic stenosis or vascular ring, vocal cord motion disorders or upper airway-intrinsic disease, or hypersensitivity pneumonitis (which can look like asthma when an in-depth history of significant inhalation exposure is overlooked). To begin, an internist or pulmonologist will ask if the symptoms seem to come and go, and if the patient can identify any particular circumstances that trigger them. They will ask about symptoms such as chronic cough, sputum production, wheezing or audible "noisy" breathing, chest tightness, and shortness of breath, as well as if symptoms increase during certain times of day or if someone with a family history of asthma or a significant atopic history. Other questions may include whether symptoms increase with illness, posture, specific exposures, activities or cold air, as well as whether symptoms are worse during a particular season.

5.1. Chronic Obstructive Pulmonary Disease (COPD)

Biomarkers are now the focus of investigation, but none are recommended as diagnostic assets for routine patient evaluation for asthma to date. Pathologically, both can manifest airway similarities, including the presence of neutrophils, eosinophils, or both, as well as bronchospasm or airway mucus glands. If, however, the consequences and treatment of chronic airway obstruction appear to have no effect on lung function improvement, it is necessary to accurately differentiate disease states. COPD can act as an independent comorbid disease, as well as co-existing with asthma, likely to cause non-reversible airflow disease when asthma exacerbation occurs that should also be considered.

Chronic obstructive pulmonary disease (COPD) is an important differential diagnosis for asthma. The characteristic features of COPD include a history of smoking, weight loss, and persistent or progressive symptoms of sputum production accompanied by cough, wheezing, and/or shortness of breath. Because the symptoms and airway obstruction that often occur in both asthma and COPD can be similar, careful clinical consideration is required to document the changes in airflow limitations which define the disease. Patients with asthma often have better post-bronchodilator flows than COPD patients. There is no evidence, however, that COPD will offer a suboptimal response to inhaled corticosteroids in general, or in combination with inhaled β2-agonists, compared with asthma in view of the response to anti-inflammatory therapy as a way to differentiate whole groups of patients with airway disease from another. Spirometry remains the primary tool for a diagnosis of obstructive lung disease, but other imaging or tissue sampling techniques can also help to confirm the diagnosis in a subset of patients with airway disease.

5.2. Heart Failure

Typical respiratory infections such as wheezing, shortness of breath and chest tightness are often associated with heart failure, but differential diagnosis should be carried out because treatment is completely different. The diagnosis of HF is based on clinical symptoms and physical findings, with conventional examinations (chest X-rays: cardiac retraction, batwing shadow, BKT, hypochondria, electrocardiogram: low volt, echo: cardiac enlargement, reduced LVEF, NTproBNP, TFG, arterial blood gases (ABG). In most cases, complaints can be managed on an outpatient basis. The main complaints of left heart failure are shortness of breath, coughing intensifies (orthopnea = paroxysmal nocturnal asthma) which can be attached to sputum. In addition, physical activity tolerance decreases. The weakness of the heart muscle shows an increase in fatigue and muscle weakness. Hyperstimulation of the heart muscle works ahead of the His-Purkinje system to progress to cardiac arrhythmia. Like drinking ginseng, patients with left heart failure tend to experience night paralysis or have to get up at night to take a deep breath.

Heart failure may be confused with asthma. Heart failure is a process that reduces myocardial function or the ability of the heart to pump blood to all parts of the body. This process is the result of an unreasonable debt between the needs and the natural ability of the heart. Acute and chronic heart failure is accompanied by chest X-rays and has left heart failure. The main symptoms and signs of left heart failure are shortness of breath, anxiety and cold,

cough, orthopnea (complaints often occur at night,
requiring the patient to hold the neck with an erect neck or
use an additional bed so that the foot is above the heart).
paralysis. The duration of the coughing during cardiac load
is also important. If over time coughing occurs, this
disorder could be caused by CPSD.

6. Treatment Guidelines for Asthma

This comprehensive guideline recommends comprehensive therapies tailored for each of the four levels of asthma. Non-pharmacological treatments that are also important include asthma action plans, trigger reduction/avoidance, and patient, family, and caregivers' asthma education. Co-managing allergic rhinitis is recommended. Patient preferences must be considered and tailored to each asthma patient's medical, social, and mental health needs. Inhaled allergen immunotherapy (A-I-T) is now recommended as an option for some patients who continue to experience symptoms and exacerbations from allergen exposure such as house dust mites or pollen. Inhaled A-I-T decreased symptom scores, as-needed SABA use, and induces allergen tolerance that persists at least 2 years after discontinuation of treatment. For patients for whom allergens are a trigger, such as aeroallergen-exposed patients with reactive airways, consider referral for allergist consultation to review desensitization options. Histamine and platelet-activating factor antagonist tablets are not recommended as monotherapy for patients with intermittent mild asthma. Long-term controller therapy is recommended for mild persistent asthma. The asthma phenotypes are noted within the guideline and may be helpful for the practitioner to predict response to therapies.

The National Asthma Education and Prevention Program 2020 asthma management guidelines are an extensive scientific research document that clinical researchers, policy makers, and many peer-reviewed published studies have contributed to. This extensive document is intended to aid clinical decision-making and to outline the treatment that is needed to change the level of asthma in the population. The guidelines are also comprehensive in their approach to managing patients of different levels of asthma control, i.e. managing asthma patients with different levels of asthma severity including intermittent, mild persistent, moderate persistent, and severe persistent asthma. They offer recommendations for managing patients with these differing levels of disease severity, pharmacological recommendations for treatment of asthma with inhaled corticosteroids of varying strengths, short-acting beta-agonists (SABA), and long-acting beta-agonists (LABA), biologics, and oral corticosteroids (OCS) including information on reducing and stopping corticosteroids. The recommendations for treating asthma at each level consist of both pharmacological and non-pharmacological interventions that are necessary to achieve and maintain control so that the impact of asthma can be minimized in the population. Familiarity with the 2020 Asthma Guideline is essential if optimal care is to be provided for asthma control.

6.1. Pharmacological Management

Currently, the pharmacological treatment of asthma is divided between two medications: medication to relieve bronchoconstriction (SABA, LABA, LAMA, oral corticosteroid) and medications to control inflammation (ICS, ICS and LABA, LTRA, theophylline, monoclonal antibody). Bronchodilator drugs also reduce cough and wheezing and assist in the elimination of inhaled allergens and irritants from the airways. Long-term management of asthma is primarily aimed at reducing airway inflammation and preventing symptoms, exacerbations, and reducing asthma mortality. Introducing daily medication from the first visit has been shown to reduce the need for subsequent medical intervention and the future risk of hospitalizations and presentations to the emergency department.

Most patients with asthma should receive bronchodilator therapy to treat symptoms when present and reduce the bronchoconstrictor response to triggers. Most patients also require anti-inflammatory medications to reduce airway inflammation and airway remodeling. The pharmacological management of asthma is one that focuses on minimizing and controlling symptoms, maintaining an optimal level of lung function, preventing acute exacerbations, providing bronchodilator relief for acute asthma, minimizing the use of rescue medication, reducing emergency-room visits and hospitalization and associated costs, and minimizing adverse effects of therapy. The preferred drug products and devices used to deliver asthma medications for this treatment are listed in the Canadian asthma guidelines. Clinicians need to know and understand the various medications available to manage asthma so that they can initiate appropriate therapy to optimize asthma control. There are patient-related factors that could impact medication selection, including patient preference, age, work experience with medications, and cost of medications.

long-term management. The goal of asthma management is to halt the symptoms from developing and helping in reducing the frequency of asthma episodes. The earlier the triggers are identified and intervention started, the better the results can be achieved in terms of healthful physical experience.

7. Asthma Action Plans

There are three components of an asthma action plan: definitions (or classifications) of symptoms based on patient-reported experiences, self-management strategies, and recommendations on when to call a healthcare provider. The self-management and provider call strategies in plans for adults revolve around the use of medications and response to medications, with the use of criteria for increasing anti-inflammatory medication becoming more standard. There is much less evidence addressing effective self-management strategies when developing plans for children. The use of plans allows patients to self-monitor their condition and take action when their asthma symptoms are not improving according to the recommendations in their plan. Regular monthly reports of an individual's asthma symptoms and lung function could be generated from a patient's action plan and allow for both individual and population-based surveillance.

Asthma action plans are a recommended best practice designed to help bridge the chasm between physicians' expert knowledge and a patient's contextual wisdom. Plans are developed collaboratively between patients and healthcare providers to provide individualized guidelines for controlling asthma symptoms and reducing the likelihood of an acute exacerbation. Plans are based on an assessment of a patient's knowledge of asthma, recognition of their unique symptoms, treatment goals, and their environmental triggers and resources.

8. Monitoring Asthma Control

The presence of persistent impairments and recurrent exacerbations indicates that treatment is not controlling asthma, and the potential for severe exacerbations and accelerated decline in lung function increase. Prevention of chronic symptoms is essential in gauging the level of control for the individual, with a 'no' response indicating the need to step up treatment. Asthma control should be reviewed regularly in patients and treatment adjusted if necessary. Assessment of control will again rely on symptoms and lung function. The continued regular treatment of chronic disease or narrowing the level of control can be avoided using a planned step-down approach. The link between type of asthma and parameters for monitoring asthma immunology is not well established, and further cross-sectional studies with a large number of subjects are required.

Regular assessment of symptoms and lung function is required to determine if treatment is controlling asthma. The more severe a patient's asthma and the more uncertain their diagnosis, the more frequent the monitoring. For those with good control, the monitoring interval should be increased. Parameters for monitoring asthma control include preventing chronic symptoms such as waking at night or experiencing breathlessness; subtle signs including the ability to engage in normal activity and exercise; the functionality of the lungs including the measurement of FEV1 percentage compared to personal best and the measurement of PEF; using a written asthma action plan for self-management; avoiding chronic use of short-acting beta-agonists; preventing cognitive, emotional, or behavior problems; reports of exacerbations causing admissions to hospital, emergency room visits, or a burst of systemic corticosteroids and any side effects experienced.

9. Emerging Technologies in Asthma Diagnosis and Treatment

Personalized medicine holds the promise of matching the right medication, at the optimal dosage and frequency to the right patient, at the right time. For asthma, this concept is particularly appealing given the vast heterogeneity in etiology and pathophysiology that often leads to variable treatment responses. There has been a significant shift in the last decade towards the development and approval of precision therapies for asthma. This new generation of medications targets specific cellular pathways underlying asthma disease heterogeneity. However, a major limitation to the success of these medications is the reliable identification of an individual's inflammatory phenotype. Clusters of asthma patients identified via omics-based data are often different from inflammatory phenotypes defined in the clinic, leading to difficulties in the translation of such tests to routine care. Moreover, while bronchoalveolar lavage and bronchial biopsy are useful tools for biomarker research, neither is feasible for diagnosis of asthma in the office or clinic. Characterization of asthma based on a single biomarker is unlikely to have more than a small to moderate impact on the diagnostic accuracy over currently available clinical assessment tools.

Within this clinical review, we focus on 9 emerging technologies aiming to reform the strategies used for asthma diagnosis and treatment. These 9 technologies were selected for their innovative and groundbreaking concepts which will drastically improve the current state of asthma testing. Some of these concepts are in their infancy and may likely never hit the market; however, electronic health records and composite biomarkers are technologies already woven into patient care. These emerging technologies could have far-reaching impacts in asthma care.

Diagnostic Tests for Asthma-Like Symptoms

1. Introduction to Asthma-Like Symptoms

It can help to identify people with asthma that present only with cough, and it is likely to be helpful in the management of people who present with asthma-like symptoms even when allergic or allergic and non-allergic inflammation is present. All the measures identify a subgroup of people with asthma-like symptoms, although the relevance of the biological samples is unknown. Thus, any isolated patient who is negative for challenge does not have diagnostic tests for asthma-like symptoms, but those who are positive have asthma-like symptoms, with a higher prevalence in those with a diagnosis of asthma versus a negative diagnosis.

Asthma and asthma-like symptoms are significant chronic respiratory diseases and major public health issues. Asthma-like symptoms refer to a new onset of wheeze, chest tightness, shortness of breath, dry cough, or phlegm not associated with the common cold, infection, or the presence of other types of airway disease. These symptoms may occur independently of asthma or may accompany the symptoms of asthma. Bronchial hyper-responsiveness (BHR), as measured by bronchial provocation tests (BPT) and bronchodilator reversibility (BDR), helps to differentiate people with asthma from those without asthma-like symptoms.

2. Importance of Diagnostic Tests

Diagnostic tests have multiple roles: (1) the probability of asthma rises proportionally as the test results increase; (2) in the interpretation of ambiguous symptoms, a normal test result allows the physician to move away from asthma and direct the patient to diagnostic alternatives; (3) in addition to other test results, positive results increase the post-test probability of asthma, and (4) it forms criteria to evaluate treatment effects (as used in diagnostic studies). It is also stressed that the panoptic diagnostic test is still not available. As a result, tests usually are complementary, not substitutes for clinical judgment. Information about a patient without various clinical characteristics is provided by the different available combinations of clinical characteristics in a given patient (of age, sex, history such as an onset of wheezing, heredity, smoking, allergy, and occupational history) and results of various diagnostic tests that are best established for asthma.

While the discussion and approaches in various parts of the world are diverse, the experts, in general, disagreed with the proposed thresholds for the definitive diagnosis of asthma as a potential response to asthma. Nonetheless, it is an essential part of the diagnostic algorithms for asthma and other disease-presentation oppositions emanating in a primary-care setting that warrants close scrutiny. Different thresholds have also been reported to exist for the reversibility of FEV1 or for lability of bronchoconstriction, both indicative of the asthma process (e.g., lability). In the

case of asthma-like symptoms, established guidelines
advise the physician to perform a diagnostic workup rather
than making a diagnosis based on symptoms alone.

3. Medical History and Physical Examination

The role of physical examination is to look for signs that suggest an alternative diagnosis and to assess indicators of asthma severity. Look for signs of heart failure in older patients. Look for conjunctivitis, signs of rhinosinusitis, systemic inflammation, and clubbing to indicate conditions that mimic asthma or have a confirmed diagnosis. In adults, wheeze due to chronic obstructive pulmonary disease usually has a slower expiratory time than patients with asthma, with reduced chest movement and signs of over-inflation. The presence, absence, and severity of asthma also have a significant relationship to inflammatory cell patterns in induced sputum. Persons who present with symptoms that are suggestive of asthma should undergo several examinations to ascertain the presence of asthma, the absence of lung diseases, and to confirm the presence of other diseases apart from asthma. Such tests are divided into eight sections and may include other tests not listed.

Physical Examination

A medical history cannot establish the diagnosis of an asthma-like symptom, but it provides a healthcare worker an opportunity to find answers to certain questions. The medical history should determine whether the breathlessness, wheezing, or cough are due to asthma or are due to an alternative diagnosis. If asthma seems probable, then the medical history should give some clue as to how the patient's asthma might respond to treatment. It is known that most successful treatment outcomes in patients with asthma have nothing to do with indicators of the severity or the relative strength of this diagnosis. In patients starting regularly inhaled corticosteroid therapy, who are already taking other treatments for asthma, the only factor that has a robust relationship with the possibility of a painful condition improving substantially is a current smoker or recent ex-smoker (> 20 pack/years).

Medical History

4. Pulmonary Function Tests

Additionally, certain parameters that relate to an increased forced expiration, compared with a slower time frame of forceful expiration, can evaluate the presence of small airway obstructions in an individual's lungs. Spirometry, with or without bronchodilator response, is used to measure some of these respiratory parameters. It is an office test and can also be used for screening. The peak flow test is a simpler office-based measurement. It has a generally higher degree of variability and is less precise than spirometry. However, it can be used to measure the presence of moderate to severe airway obstructions, identify a change in a subject's status in the office, or monitor the impact upon the patient of avoidance from damaged airways. Flow volume loop measurement gives a graphical description of forced-inhaled and forced-exhaled spirometry measurements. This is helpful, as it identifies the existence of extrathoracic upper and/or intrathoracic central airway obstruction, the existence of vocal cord movements, and strength of expiratory muscle control. A complete discussion of pulmonary function and bronchial provocation tests can be found in the ATS requirements for diagnostic tests.

Various tests to assess lung function are available to help measure lung volumes, lung capacities, rates associated with lung volumes, and the flow rate of air in and out of the lungs. Results from these tests can determine the amount of air an individual is breathing in and out of the lungs, as well as the efficiency of the mechanics associated with the respiratory process. Total lung capacity, or the total volume of air in the lungs when an individual inhales maximally, is known as one of the most common parameters. When lung volume tests are administered, data can provide physicians with an indication as to whether or not the results are abnormal.

4.1. Spirometry

The spirometer measures the following: a. Forced expiratory volume in one second (FEV1): the amount of air expired in the first second of a forced exhalation. This is followed by the total volume of air, known as forced vital capacity (FVC), that is expired. The FEV1/FVC ratio is sometimes used to assist in diagnosis: a value of less than or equal to 0.70 is indicative of obstructive airflow limitation consistent with asthma. b. Peak expiratory flow (PEF): the highest airflow rate that is achieved during a forced expiration starting from full inspiration. c. Forced expiratory flow (FEF25-75% or FEF75): the average flow rate at a certain level of lung volume in the middle of a forced expiration. d. Slow vital capacity (SVC): the volume of air that usually follows the maximum inspiration.

Spirometry is the measurement of the volume of air that a person can exhale and the time this takes. It is a reliable diagnostic test performed in the day-to-day clinical setting. The results of spirometry are reproducible and are an important tool in assessing respiratory disease severity. This test is also used to monitor the improvement in symptoms and lung function with treatment. The procedure is performed with a spirometer, a compressed air source, a nose clip, a mouthpiece, and a recorder. Before the test, people are guided correctly on how to blow forcefully into the mouthpiece to obtain reliable results. Portable electronic spirometers have a digital display that shows the results immediately after the test.

4.2. Peak Flow Test

Disadvantages and Limitations to Using the Test: The test only measures one aspect of lung function, and so may not reflect the full picture. Even in cases of better lung function, a patient may still experience symptoms. In certain conditions such as nocturnal asthma, cough variant asthma and during the initial stages of asthma (due to the condition being brought about through an infection rather than an allergic trigger), the test result may still read as being relatively normal in patients who experience ongoing mild and problematic symptoms. The test may also show a 'good' reading if the individual has taken their (improving) reliever treatment prior to the test.

The peak flow test uses a device known as the peak flow meter in order to assess an individual's maximum speed of exhalation, with the graph plotted from the test results representing the rate of air flow as exhalation takes place. Peak flow monitoring can provide the doctor with an objective method of gaining information with respect to the function of the airways, and therefore useful for tracking the progress of the condition when diagnosed (recovery or worsening). It is also used by 30% of doctors to form part of a patient's asthma action plan, which is designed to provide asthma sufferers with a guide as to when their medication may be giving less control over symptoms, and highlighting when emergency assistance would be required.

5. Imaging Tests

Because asthma can look like other diseases, it is often difficult to diagnose without checking your lung function. In some cases, if the patient is having an asthma attack and their oxygen level is decreased, a chest X-ray might be ordered to make sure there is not another cause of decreased oxygen. If the patient has new symptoms, like weight loss or not feeling well, a chest X-ray might be ordered to check for another underlying chest infection or problem. If there is doubtful asthma that doesn't respond to treatment or isn't getting better as expected, or newly diagnosed asthma in adults, some experts recommend that other tests be done to rule out other diseases. Usually if they are done, they are only done once. The tests can include a chest X-ray, sinus CT, and upper airway evaluation. A rare form of asthma can be seen on a lung CT-scan when the large airways have been narrowed by swelling (eosinophilic bronchitis). However, in most people with difficult asthma a chest X-ray or CT-scan won't show very much.

Some patients might have a chest X-ray ordered during an asthma attack. A chest X-ray can show complications of asthma in the chest. This might happen more with people who are older or have other serious lung diseases. Sometimes a contrast X-ray, also called an angiogram or angiography, is done to make sure that the arteries in your lungs are open and healthy. This might need to be done if you are preparing for lung surgery or if you have been diagnosed with pulmonary hypertension. A chest X-ray can show a few common signs of asthma in severe cases, but how the lungs look doesn't tell your doctor if you have airway inflammation or not.

X-rays are not often useful for diagnosing asthma, but they may be ordered to check for other lung diseases. One condition that shows up on X-ray is pneumonia. Viral infections combined with asthma increase the risk for pneumonia. Patients with chronic sinusitis are also at increased risk of pneumonia. Some drugs given for pneumonia treatment can worsen asthma. An X-ray can also show your doctor other conditions that look like asthma.

5.1. Chest X-ray

A chest X-ray is typically the first imaging test used to help diagnose wheezing, coughing, chest tightness, shortness of breath, and disturbance in sleep consistent with asthma. X-rays of the neck and head may also be employed. Lachman recommends a CX-ray of the sternum and upper abdominal organs should be included in the initial evaluation in adults to rule out GERD or postnasal flow. Pulmonary cystic fibrosis should be included in the differential diagnosis of airway obstruction, chronic cough, or wheezing from the study published by Yamasaki. Allergic Bronchopulmonary Aspergillosis should be in the differential diagnosis of nocturnal asthma and/or postnasal flow and chronic unexplained cough in children due to chest pain and shortness of breath, previously published suggestions for adults. Certain diagnoses have different CX-ray abnormality frequencies that make the value of CX-ray different in an individual with established chronic asthma compared to an obstacle.

Chest X-ray (CXR) is a widely used non-invasive technique for imaging the chest. A posterior-anterior (PA) view is most commonly obtained by the CX-ray technologist. Additional oblique, lateral, and apico-basal views (carried out when the patient's condition allows it) provide orthogonal information useful in detailed assessment. CXR is a quick and reliable technique to secure the airway, oxygenate, and ventilate the patient. Plain CXR provides anatomical information of the thoracic cage and respiratory system with sufficient detail to give an impression of the presence or absence of focal or diffuse abnormalities. In a restricted number of cases, it allows a definitive diagnosis or reduces the diagnosis to a limited number of possibilities. If CXR is indicative of small airway involvement in the cervico-thoracal area, other more detailed imaging studies are required (e.g., HRCT lungs).

5.2. CT Scan

Asthma: Low-attenuation areas in the lungs could be a sign of inflammation. Bronchiolitis: Inflammation and mucus causing airway blockage are visible. Bronchiectasis: This is a destructive lung condition, in which the larger airways in the lungs become damaged and widen. 'Flesh-eating' necrotizing pneumonia: A very severe form of pneumonia, in which lung tissue dies, causes pockets of gas to form. Atelectasis: A small area of the lung could collapse. Recurrent pneumonia: A pocket of pus in the lung. Pulmonary embolism: A clot in the lung. Other lung/respiratory conditions can also be diagnosed.

When you breathe in, you can reach your optimum lung volume (a process known as inspiration). A good CT image requires you to take a deep breath and hold it for a few seconds. While this may make it easier for you to see your lungs, some people find it difficult. The scan exposes you to a small quantity of radiation. Modern CT scanners use new designs and minimize your radiation exposure. You can go back to your usual activities when your CT scan is done. There are no known side effects. Although only a specialist radiologist can provide an exact diagnosis from a CT scan, it can provide useful information about:

A CT (computerized tomography) scan provides detailed cross-sectional images of your body in layers, rather than in just one 3D picture. This lets your doctor see your lungs in more detail than with a chest x-ray. It only takes a few seconds to have a CT scan; however, it takes time to construct the precise image.

6. Allergy Testing

Performing at-home immediate hypersensitivity penicillin skin testing is not recommended as it carries a risk of severe cutaneous adverse reactions, such as anaphylaxis or Stevens-Johnson syndrome/toxic epidermal necrolysis. The at-home controlled ingestion challenge also has a very high rate of anaphylaxis and should be standardized if conducted. Alternatively, skin prick tests and either serum-specific IgE random wheat extract (as is available in Korean bakeries), or better yet, wheat proteins, such as wheat omega-5 gliadin or lipid transfer protein (such as Pru p 3), should be used to assess for possible gluten-containing food allergy/intolerance.

Skin prick tests (SPT) are the most common type of trim cut tests and have been used in many of the studies we have already mentioned. Prick to prick is a modification of the SPT that has been used to directly assess for allergen sensitization in fruits and vegetables that are not commercially available. In an evaluable skin prick test, the sum of the two perpendicular measurements of the wheal in millimeters yields a result. If the positive (histamine) control result is not > 3 millimeters, the test result is non-evaluable. Skin-tip tests are contraindicated for many dermatologic conditions. Assessments can also be affected by the lack of skin reactivity in healthy volunteers, the subjective interpretation of the test results, and the arbitrary cut-off for interpreting positivity.

7. Blood Tests

- Complete blood count (CBC): This test measures the number of white blood cells, reticulocytes (a measure of new red cell production), and evaluates the number of red blood cells, including volume, hematocrit, and hemoglobin concentration. - Eosinophil count: This test measures the number of eosinophils circulating in the blood. Eosinophils are a white blood cell involved in allergic and immune responses. - Eosinophil cationic protein (ECP): ECP is a protein primarily present within eosinophils. A small amount is released from an eosinophil's granules during degranulation, making it a marker of eosinophil activity. It may aid in the diagnosis of asthma. Both increased and decreased ECP levels have been seen in asthma patients. - Immunocap Specific IgEs: This test measures the presence of specific antibodies (immunoglobulin E) to common allergens (e.g. dust mite, dog). Higher IgE results are associated with a likelihood of allergy; however, they cannot rule out asthma or allergy just because the results are normal. - Fractional exhaled nitric oxide (FcNO): This blood test measures inflammation in your lungs. Nitric oxide is a gas made by cells in your body. Elevated FeNO is not specific for asthma and can be related to other lung diseases and conditions.

Blood tests are done to check other conditions that may be related to asthma-like symptoms, such as increased production of white blood cells (eosinophils). There are no specific tests that can strongly prove that you have asthma.

However, these blood tests can help your doctor figure out if your symptoms are caused by asthma or might be related to something else.

8. Sputum Eosinophil Count

Several cells can be assessed in sputum. These cells include macrophages, neutrophils, eosinophils, CD4 cells, and CD8 cells. In subjects with asthma, typically, greater than 3% sputum eosinophils are considered increased. Sputum eosinophils are a weak biomarker for other airway eosinophil phenotypes. However, sputum eosinophils are a useful biomarker for identifying responders to corticosteroids. The interest in sputum cell counts relates to a molecular phenotyping of the asthma syndrome. Based on this concept, increased concentrations of eosinophils, neutrophils, and lymphocytes in sputum are associated with distinct types of asthma. Eosinophilic predominant phenotypes respond to corticosteroids. Treatment of eosinophilic sputum with an inhaled corticosteroid can reduce asthma exacerbation rates in comparison to the placebo group. Guiding medical treatment with sputum eosinophils also decreases asthma symptoms in comparison to inhaled corticosteroids (ICS) step-care treatment. Anti-interleukin (IL)-5 with eosinophilic phenotype decreases asthma exacerbations compared to placebo. It also reduces cough and sputum weight. Sputum investigations are invasive. Perseverating through coughing increases the amount of sputum but also the amount of oropharyngeal sputum, increasing eosinophilia. Greater than 0.25×10^6 sputum eosinophils/ml, representing 3% of total cytology sheet eosinophils, is considered an increase. A sputum eosinophil count greater than 3 to 4% has the highest positive likelihood ratio (PLR) for identifying therapeutic responders.

Sputum eosinophil count helps in assessing airway inflammation in subjects with asthma-like symptoms. Sputum guiding treatment towards a pharmacological reduction in eosinophilic airway inflammation results in a reduction in exacerbation rate, a decrease in oral steroid course number, fewer chronic obstructive airway disease (COAD) hospital admissions, a higher asthma control questionnaire score, and an increase in health-related quality of life. However, direct surgical intervention may be limited in people with asthma-like symptoms. With this in mind, this review will focus on investigations with sputum eosinophils rather than investigations directly associated with asthma.

9. Bronchoprovocation Testing

Bronchoprovocation tests provide information about several critical aspects of airway biology, but current literature of citations includes only the most relevant citations that can be easily and quickly found, which essentially includes information from the US FDA Summary Basis of Approval and ADVERSE REACTIONS - section (from Insert Label), and more complete information from the DailyMed website and the Manufacturer's Package Insert. This is to establish that the drug or chemical being added to the list causes airway constriction in at least some persons, and is generally an asthma drug with a sulfite or a food additive (for example, metabisulfite in fruit products). Raising baseline airways resistance (decreasing FEV1) by some technique (an aluminum or mannitol powder) and then inhaling the agent and measuring the response.

Bronchoprovocation tests (also called stimuli, challenges, or agents) involve techniques for inducing airway constriction in order to determine the presence or absence of asthma-like symptoms in patients with normal lung function when they are not wheezing. Most tests can be used in older children (as at 6-7 years), adolescents, and adults, can be standardized by giving different standard concentrations to the next highest concentrations in person, and have a well-established CPT code for billing. Results are reported as the concentration or dose of the agent needed to reduce FEV1 by 20%, known as the marker for a positive test. Some test results predict the development of wheezing on challenge better than others, and some may have greater test-retest reliability (reproducibility) giving better diagnostic information.

10. Exhaled Nitric Oxide Test

Measurement of nitric oxide (NO) levels is different from conventional tests for asthma because it measures inflammation or the underlying abnormality of the airways, rather than measuring functional change in the airways (for example, obstruction of airflow or bronchospasm). In children, the test is better than some other easy-to-obtain tests when there are co-morbid conditions such as seasonal symptoms which may complicate the interpretation of tests for other conditions. Furthermore, the measurement of FeNO in breath is less unpleasant to obtain, less time-consuming, less expensive, and easier to use than measurement of inflammatory cells in the blood (phlebotomy) or sputum. It can be used in the clinic, by primary care-based healthcare providers (nurse or physician), or non-healthcare professionals. The test can be performed on all age groups.

The exhaled nitric oxide (FeNO) test places the person in a sitting position with minimal upper body movement and inhales to near total lung capacity, followed by a near total lung capacity exhaled breath through a filter and chemiluminescence-based analyzer interface equipped for online nitric oxide (NO) assessment. One technique is to inhale purified, NO-free, or NO-dilute air, and the NO concentration is monitored at the end of the exhaled air inspiration. A therapeutic NO exhalation response is good evidence for adherence to the defined end-exhalation ventilation delivery procedure and is predictive for clinically significantly improved asthma outcomes (as indicated by response to a trial of corticosteroid). A statistically significantly different NO level is present in patients with asthma compared with patients with no asthma. The test is useful for monitoring treatment and detecting relapse when the patient is withdrawing successfully from corticosteroids; a rise in nitric oxide may be one of the first indicators that inflammation is returning.

11. Bronchoscopy

Bronchoscopy should be considered in patients in whom other investigations have failed to identify an alternative explanation for airflow obstruction. It may be useful in patients with asthma who present with pulmonary symptoms suggestive of other disease, including those with focal or progressive symptoms, atypical malformations from the time of diagnosis (e.g., infiltrates, hemoptysis, lobar collapse), suspected complications from asthma therapies including bronchiectasis, patients with occupational asthma with atypical features, and hemoptysis thought to be related to asthma. Although bronchoscopy plays some part in the evaluation of complex problems thought to be due to asthma, it should not be the de facto investigation but rather one that is considered in a relative minority of patients.

Bronchoscopy is a medical procedure where a fiber-optic tube about the thickness of a pencil is passed through the mouth and into the lungs. The procedure enables the physician to look at the airways and lung tissue directly, which makes it a "gold standard" for definitions and locating of abnormalities as well as the extent of disease. Bronchoscopy is not routinely used as a diagnostic tool for asthma, especially for those whose symptoms are mild or well controlled with medication. However, people with persistent symptoms may have underlying conditions such as compression due to tumors, foreign bodies, or lung infection, which in some cases a bronchoscopy is helpful to diagnose. It has been estimated that flexible bronchoscopy leads to a new diagnosis in 1.2% to 34% of adult asthmatics and may help guide their therapy.

12. Other Potential Tests

Tests of allergy-associated inflammation are additive in most circumstances. Besides blood tests for total IgE and eosinophils (typically normal in asthma without exacerbation), one may request blood levels of allergic antibodies (IgE) to specific classes of antigens, the in vitro peri reaction to antigens, and a skin prick test to transfer the antigens to a primarily cutaneous and inflamed condition before checking for allergic inflammation. Exhaled nitric oxide is a post-bringing test to measure inflammation in the bronchi. It is indicated when a clinician must verify post-bringing to broncho-reactive drugs that there is underlying allergic inflammation in the bronchi, as a cause of respiratory complaints such as exercise-related asthma, post-infectious cough, or the like. Exhaled nitric oxide can be induced by the allergen that is mechanically brought below the bifurcation of the trachea, or from the genetic materials of the inhaled agents that are brought to the innated immunity of human epithelium. In its chemical form, it has an affinity to be a morning chemical to oxidize. In medical assessment, the normal value to exclude an algorithmic way is 17.5 ppm or 25 ppb. The skill of performing a diurnal patch is to exclude non-voxel environmental or occupational factors.

Besides those covered in the first 10 sections of this document, there are a few additional tests that may be considered based on the scenario. They should be understood as tests that we may consider, depending on certain clinical scenarios, and not as absolute indications. There are many different clinical scenarios when a diagnostic test with soft indications becomes undoubtedly indicated. These additional tests are far from being part of the diagnostic routine. The first gold standard test should have been sufficient for a diagnosis of the asthma phenotype in most scenarios.

13. Preparing for Diagnostic Tests

• Bronchial Challenge Test Duration: On the day of the test, you need to allow at least 2-3 hours for the entire process. Dietary/Fluid restrictions: There are some foods (and medications) you will need to stay clear of and some over-the-counter and prescription medications you will need to stop taking for a short period allowing the bronchial challenge value to return to normal, particularly if it's been used to manage asthma effectively before. Make sure this has been addressed with your doctor prior to commencing the test. What to bring: Please remember to bring all the asthma medications you would usually use on a regular basis.

• CT Scans Duration: On the day you have the test, you'll be in the radiology department for about 20-30 minutes, or longer if you need the contrast liquid to be given during the test. Dietary/Fluid restrictions: For some tests, you will be asked to consume liquid, have a specific diet, or stop eating for a certain period in order to prepare. What to bring: A CT scan is a painless test and you will not need to bring anything with you, except any papers or clips that a doctor may have given you for the test centre.

• Sputum Induction Duration: On the day you have the test, the whole process will take about 2 hours. Dietary/Fluid restrictions: To help produce a good sample of sputum, do not eat or drink anything except water for at least three hours before the test; take any routine asthma medications. What to bring: Please remember to wear loose, comfortable clothing, and you may want to bring a book, some music, or a puzzle to help pass the time.

14. Understanding Test Results

NITRIC OXIDE IN EXHALED BREATH (FeNO50) - This measures the amounts of nitric oxide (NO) gas that a person exhales. It only measures the amount of NO that is being produced by the lining (epithelium) of the lower airway (alveoli). It has been extensively reviewed in previous chapters. REFERENCE RANGE: Complete exhalation of air into the analyzer, and the results show an exhaled nitric oxide level of 1-30ppb, which is generally acceptable. A high level of FeNO50 in the expired air (over 30ppb) generally indicates that a patient's lower airway (alveoli) is inflamed.

The diagnostic process for asthma-like symptoms includes several tests which are used to determine the presence of an active allergic or other adverse reactions. An understanding of the implications of these tests is critical for both you and your healthcare provider. Presented below are the allergy and physiological tests that you may have had. There is information on what the test measures, the results you may have received, and the implications of those results. These tests comprise the Aerocrine System. Generally, our tests are performed simultaneously with allergy tests. As we do not test for allergies, the test results presented here are interpreted on the basis of your symptoms according to the PC appearance. However, should you be tested for allergies in the future, and test positive, you may be co-presenting with basal nitric oxide and bronchial hyperreactivity as a result of the PC test.

15. Common Misconceptions and FAQs

Could I have specialist tests, such as skin prick tests, to tell me what is causing my symptoms? Nasal nitric oxide can be performed at the discretion of the specialist if they believe there is a possibility the patient has a condition other than classical diagnostic testing for asthma. This test is not available in a primary care setting and is not generally available in every country. Allergy testing might be useful to diagnose people with a condition called allergic bronchopulmonary mycosis, however this condition requires other diagnostic tests to be confirmed.

A common misconception is that it is not possible to perform tests on young children. Whilst spirometry cannot be performed on children under the age of five years, younger children can be diagnosed with symptoms alone or by assessing how they respond to the use a reliever medication do.

Another concern commonly expressed by patients is: I can't afford to have any tests. Are tests essential? No. Contrary to this misconception, diagnostic tests are not essential. In some situations, diagnostic tests are impractical, contraindicated, or not applicable. Diagnostic testing must be interpreted alongside a detailed and comprehensive clinical evaluation. Testing should be deferred or repeated if measurement circumstances are not as per the international guidelines for spirometry.

Another frequently asked question is: My doctor has previously told me I don't need any tests if my symptoms can be controlled by my reliever inhaler. Is this correct? No. This is a misconception. Diagnostic tests provide information about lung function that can help an individual evaluate the underlying mechanisms that might be causing their asthma-like symptoms. Ultimately, this can help to guide patients' treatment plans.

There are a lot of conflicting messages regarding the use of diagnostic tests for people with asthma-like symptoms. This has often resulted in negative impacts on the health and wellbeing of patients. A frequently asked question is: What diagnostic tests are suitable for a person with asthma-like symptoms? The best diagnostic test for a person with asthma-like symptoms measures their current level of lung function using spirometry. This includes a simple test such as the forced expiratory volume in one second (FEV1) or the ratio of forced expiratory volume in one second to forced vital capacity (FEV1/FVC). If lung function levels are low, repeat testing with a bronchodilator (reliever) inhaler should be performed.

Here we address frequent questions and common misconceptions.